DIY Celebrity Haircuts

Get a Celebrity Hairstyle

Without The Expensive Salon Price!

Written and Illustrated by
NANCY HARRINGTON

DISCLAIMER

Best efforts for accuracy and completeness have been made in the creation of this book. However, no representations or warranties with respect to its accuracy and completeness, nor any implied warranty of merchantability or fitness for a particular purpose is made. The advice and suggestions contained herein may not be suitable for your situation. Consult with a professional where appropriate.

COPYRIGHTED MATERIAL

CONTENTS

About This Book 4

Preparation 6

What You'll Need 7

Two Easy-to-Learn DIY Haircutting Techniques 8

Step One – Cutting the Back 9

Step Two – Cutting the Long Side 15

Step Three – Cutting the Short Side 19

Step Four – Cutting Spikes 23

Step Five – Shaping 27

Maintenance 32

Five Minute Refresher 33

Determining Facial Shapes 37

The Importance of Bangs 47

Matching Skin Tone to Hair Color 51

Tips for Keeping Your Hair Looking Great
   (and Saving Money Too!) 53

Inspirational Hairstyles 55

ABOUT THIS BOOK

This book contains the SECRETS needed to get started on your way to saving time and money in just one day!

You will learn two NEW simple techniques to cutting and maintaining your own hair.

With many clear illustrations and easy to follow instructions, you will be able to cut your own hair in no time!

You can do this! I am not a hairdresser. Never have been. But I have been cutting my own hair for years and yes, ladies, even my untrusting husband's hair. I've taught many of my friends to cut their own hair and they encouraged me to share this in a quick easy-to-follow DIY book.

My focus in writing this book was to help put people in control of their time, money and appearance. And you WILL save lots of money!

This does not require expensive tools. I will tell you exactly what you need and at an affordable price.

It felt so good when I helped my friends learn to cut their own hair. I know this book can help you too. Many of us have talents we don't take advantage of. Think of what yours are and pass them along to help others.

This book can be used in two ways:

1. If, after reading the book completely, you feel confident and comfortable with the process, you can get started right away!

2. If you don't yet feel confident enough to cut your own hair, you may opt to have your hairdresser cut your hairstyle for you. Then with the instructions in the book you can maintain your hairstyle by following Steps 1-5. Also, take advantage of the Five-Minute Refresher section. Soon you will be comfortable enough to complete the hairstyle yourself.

PREPARATION

As with any successful project the key is preparation. Follow the instructions carefully.

Before you start your haircut, you need to remove all product residues from your hair. This will help your hair to have more volume.

Wash your hair with your usual shampoo and rinse. Pour a small amount of an astringent into your hair and comb it through. Follow immediately with a thorough rinse.

Blow dry your hair while shaking your head and running your fingers through it. Your hair should reveal its natural part and the direction that it naturally falls in. This is very important. Do not try to force you hair into a direction in which it does not naturally grow. Hair falling naturally into place is the basis for a good haircut.

NOTE

Cut your hair when it is completely dry unless otherwise instructed.

WHAT YOU'LL NEED

4" Straight Scissor

4" Thinning Scissor

 Small Hand Mirror

Styling Brush

Comb

Clips

Boar Bristle Brush

Razor

Fragrance Free Lotion

Astringent

You do not have to spend top dollar for these items. I have used very reasonably priced tools and gotten great results. If you are more comfortable with purchasing high end materials then by all means do so.

TWO EASY TO LEARN DIY HAIRCUTTING TECHNIQUES

The following pages outline two easy to follow DIY basic haircutting techniques:

1. **CUTTING** – For cutting use a straight scissor.
2. **SHAPING** – For shaping use a thinning scissor.

You will have more control when using a shorter scissor with four inch blades.

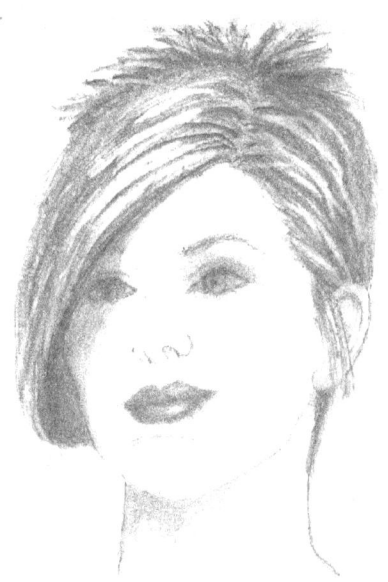

I am using the Kate Gosselin hairstyle as a learning tool. After completing steps 1-5 you will have learned the two basic DIY haircutting techniques to easily cut this hairstyle or others that you may choose. See the many combinations that are available at the end of the book.

STEP ONE

Cutting the Back

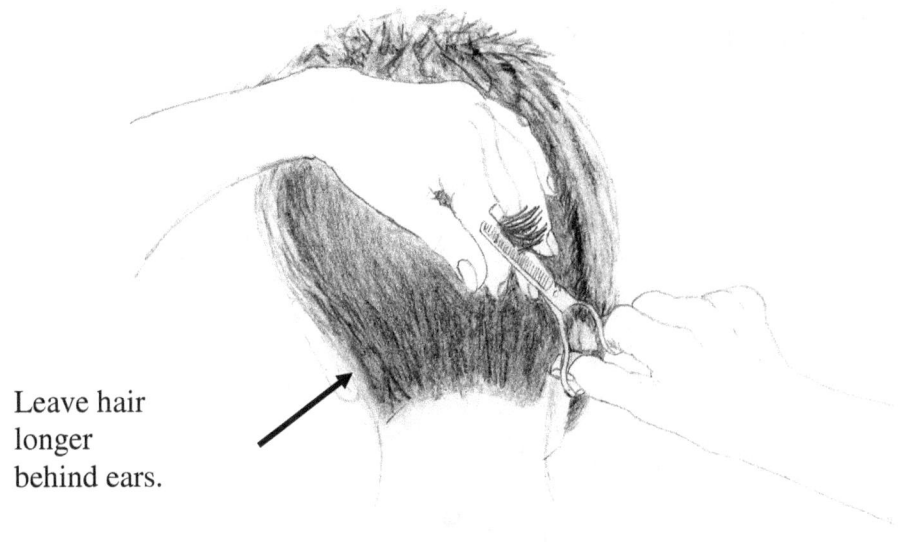

Leave hair longer behind ears.

Figure 1-1

NOTE

Cut hair when dry unless otherwise noted.

NOTE

Throughout this book you will notice that the illustrations will show the hairstyle as completed. This is done to show the direction in which we are going. It is important that you cut only what is being described in each section.

Grasp hair between two fingers as illustrated in *Figure 1-1*. Use of a thinning scissor will help prevent "cut marks" in the back of your hair. Using the thinning scissor, cut along the top of your fingers (use the depth of your fingers as your depth gauge). Notice how I have shaped the hair to the back of the ears as in *Figure 1-2*. Also note how I change the position of my hands as I move around the back of my head.

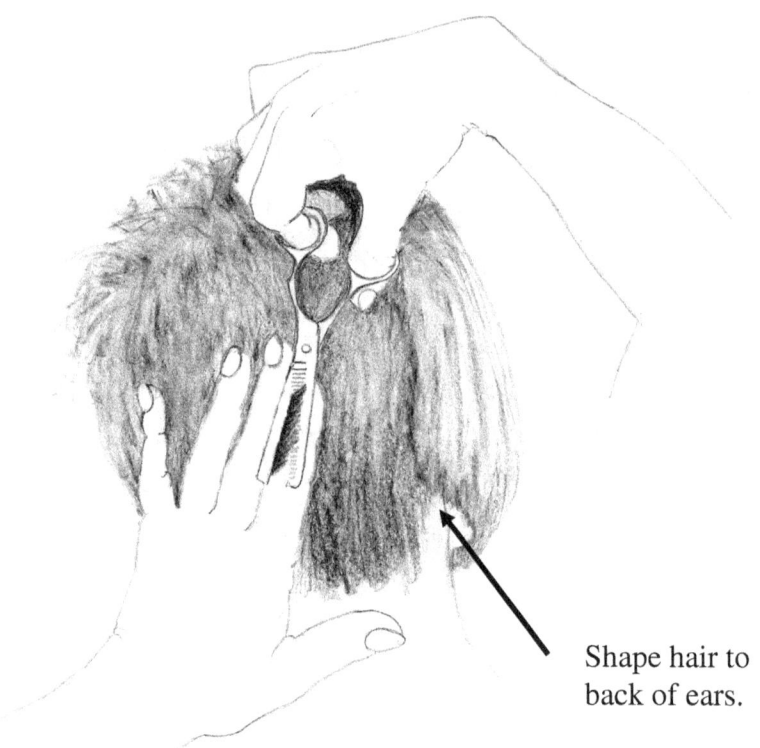

Shape hair to back of ears.

Figure 1-2

In *Figure 1-1* and *Figure 1-2*, I am not using a mirror; therefore I start cutting at the neckline and work my way towards the top. Occasionally stop and check in the mirror. Follow the shape of the short hair intersecting with the long hair. See *Figure 1-3*.

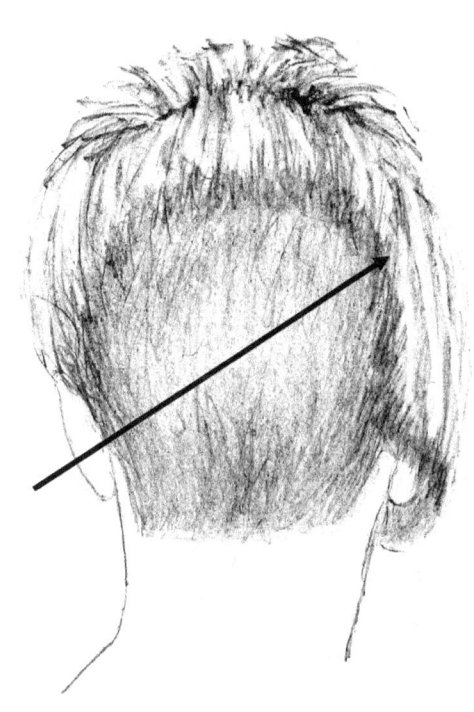

Short hair
intersecting with
long hair.

Figure 1-3

Remember, if you cut your hair when it is wet, it will "shrink" after drying. Make sure you cut a little longer than the finished length that you want to compensate. You can always cut more. Always cut hair dry unless otherwise noted.

Wet the back of your hair and comb down against the neck (*Figure 1- 4*). Using your hand mirror and straight scissor, cut hair as illustrated in *Figure 1-4 Before.*

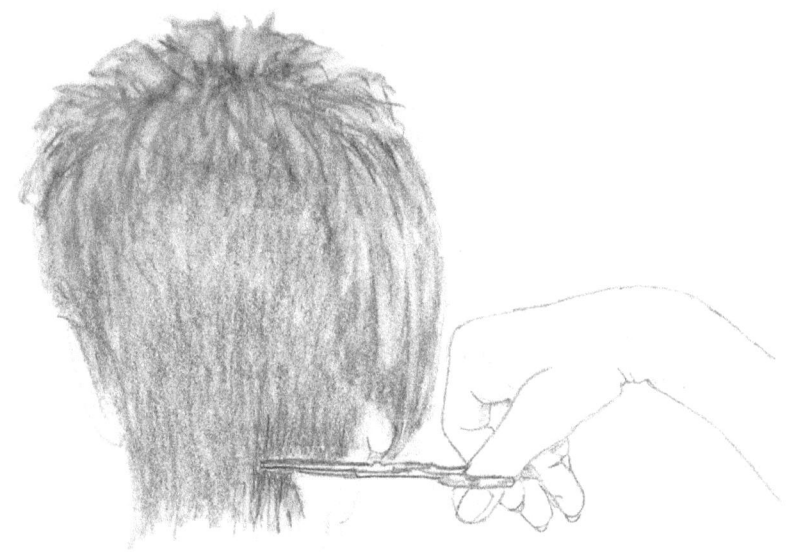

Figure 1-4 Before

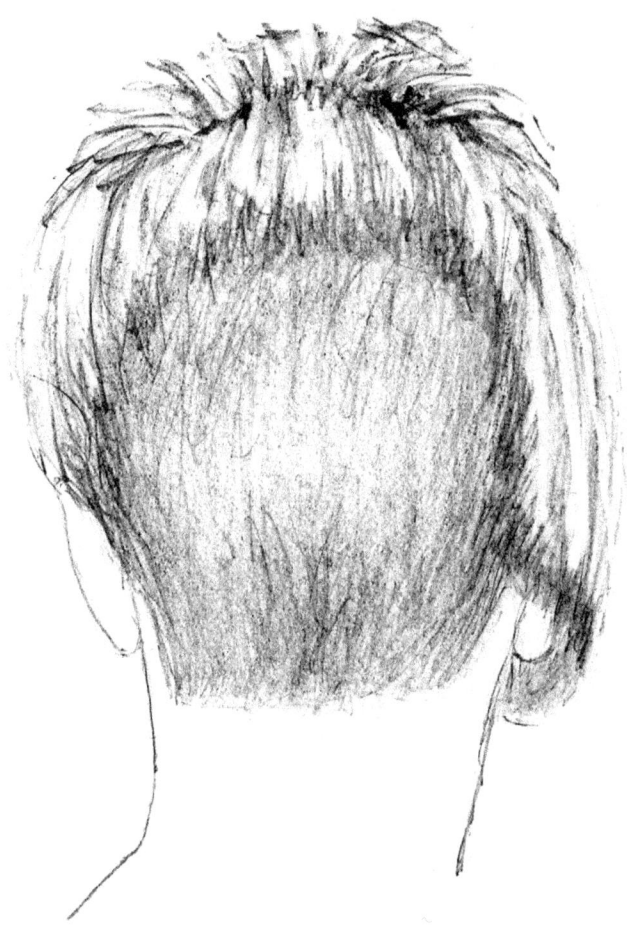

Figure 1-4 After

Apply fragrance-free lotion (to prevent irritation), to back of the neck and shave neck hair as illustrated in *Figure 1-5*.

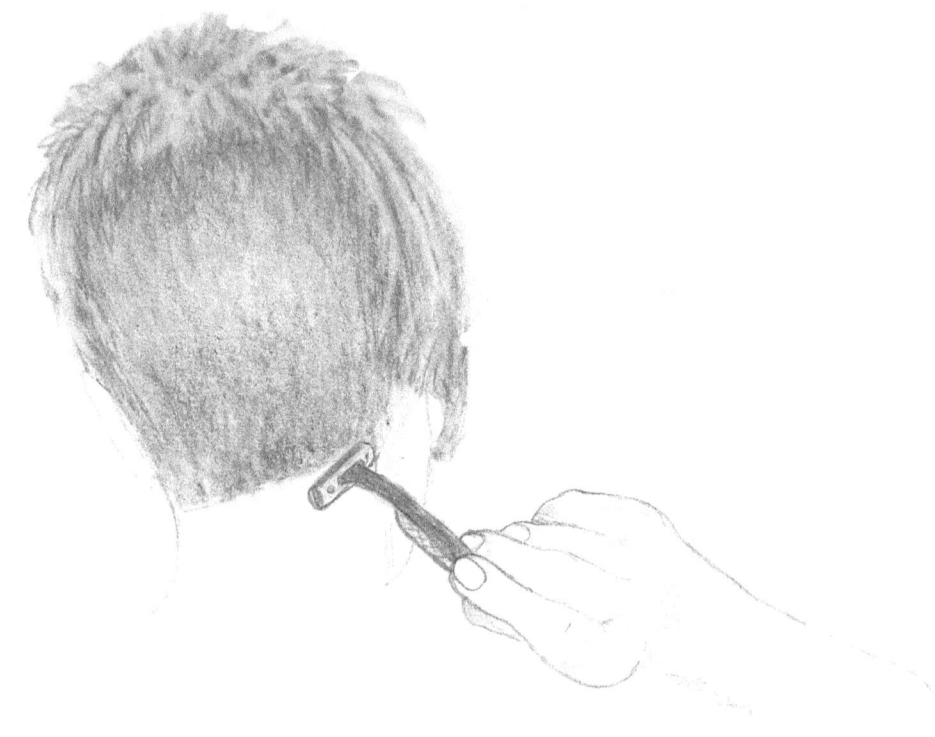

Figure 1-5

STEP 2
Cutting the Long Side

NOTE

Remember, if you cut your hair when it is wet, it will "shrink" after drying. Make sure you cut a little longer than the finished length you want, to compensate. You can always cut more.

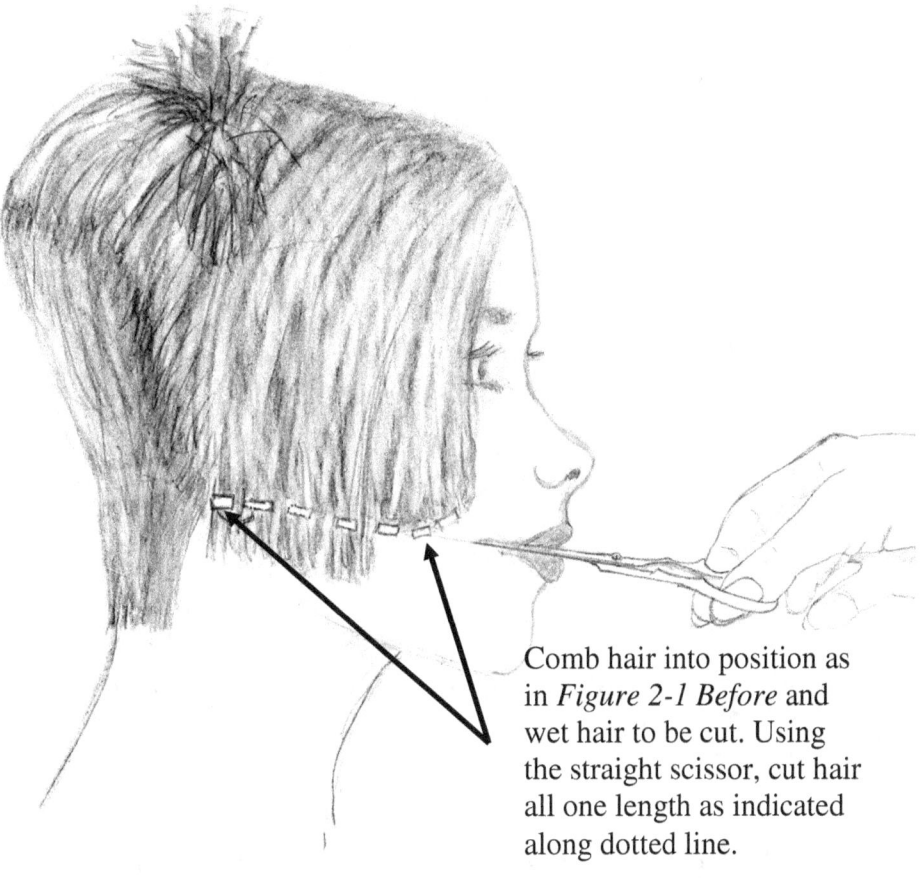

Comb hair into position as in *Figure 2-1 Before* and wet hair to be cut. Using the straight scissor, cut hair all one length as indicated along dotted line.

Figure 2-1 Before

Once your hair has dried it should fall to within your lip line while slightly showing the earlobe as shown in *Figure 2-1 After*.

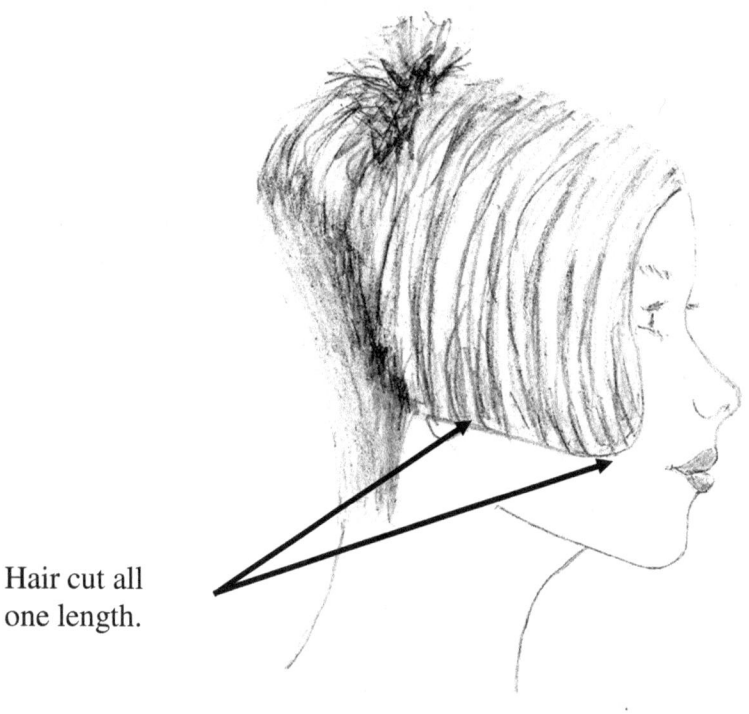

Hair cut all one length.

Figure 2-1 After

After the hair has been cut as in *Figure 2-1 After*, the next step is illustrated in *Figure 2-2 Before*.

Part hair and clip it on top of your head as in *Figure 2-2 Before*. Wet the hair to be cut and use the straight scissor to cut off one quarter inch. At this time gently intersect the side hair with the back hair.

Part hair
and clip it
on top of
head.

Cut hair to
intersect
side hair
with back
hair.

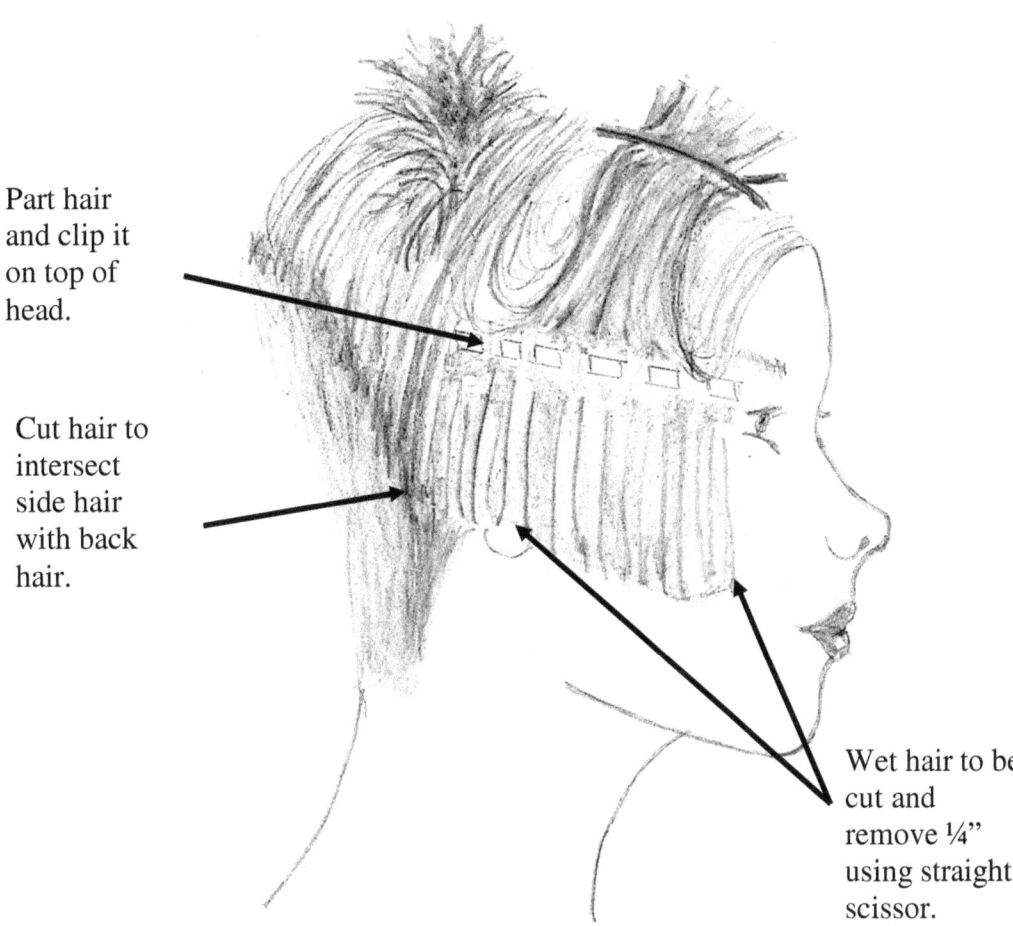

Wet hair to be
cut and
remove ¼"
using straight
scissor.

Figure 2-2 Before

NOTE

Cutting the hair one-quarter inch shorter underneath will encourage the top hair to turn under.

Figure 2-2 After shows the finished look after successfully completing Step 2.

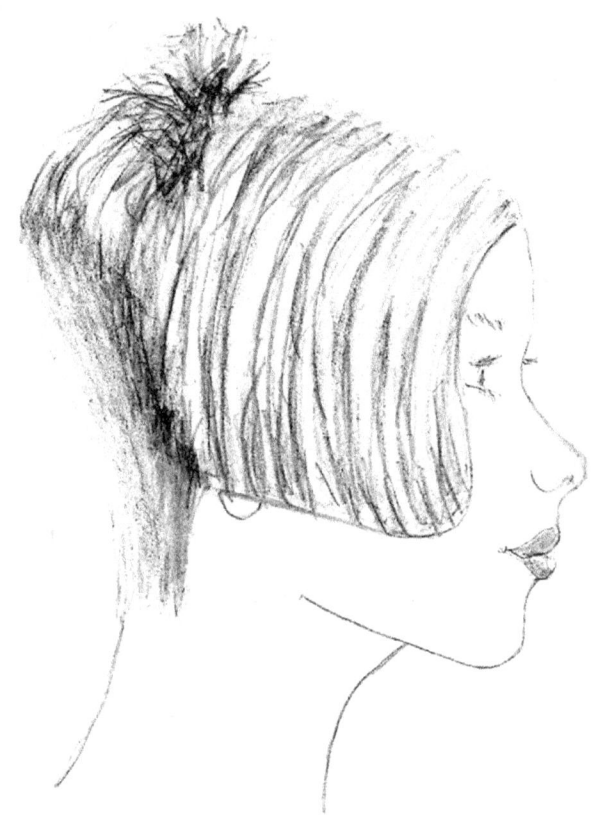

Figure 2-2 After

Run your fingers through your hair while shaking your head. This will encourage your hairstyle to naturally show itself.

STEP THREE

Cutting the Short Side

NOTE

Remember, if you cut your hair when it is wet, it will "shrink" after drying. Make sure you cut it a little longer than the finished length you want, to compensate. You can always cut more.

Cut hair long enough to cover top of ear & long enough to stay behind your ear.

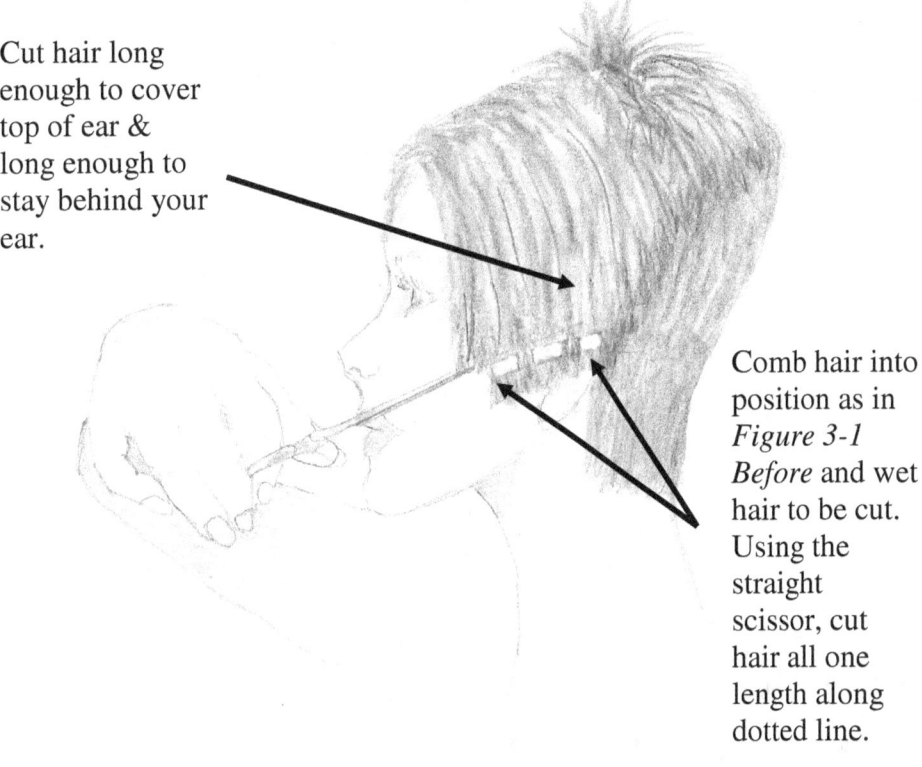

Comb hair into position as in *Figure 3-1 Before* and wet hair to be cut. Using the straight scissor, cut hair all one length along dotted line.

Figure 3-1 Before

Once your hair has dried it should be long enough to cover the top of your ear as shown in *Figure 3-1 After.*

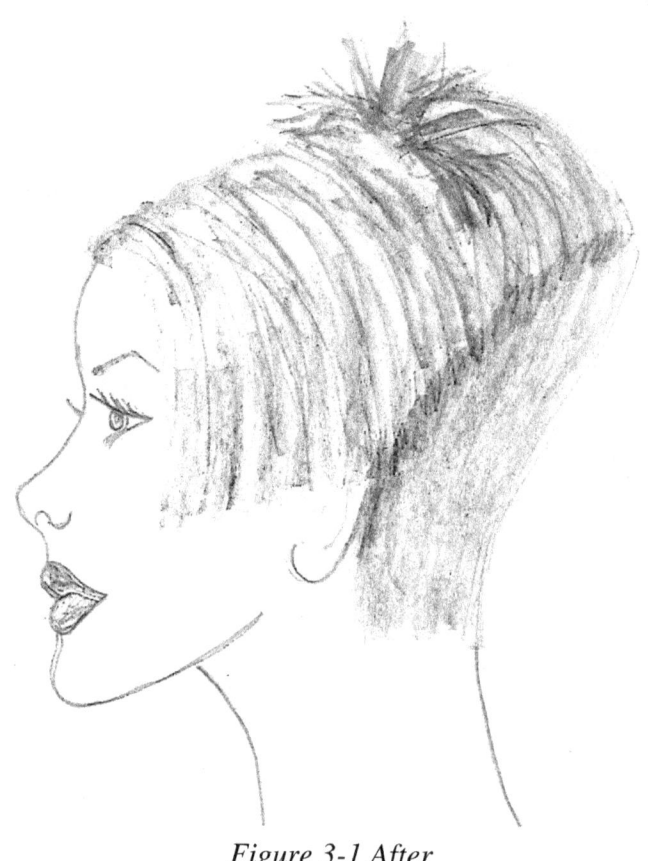

Figure 3-1 After

After hair has been cut as in *Figure 3-1 After*, the next step is illustrated in *Figure 3-2 Before.*

Part hair and clip on top of head as in *Figure 3-2 Before*. Wet the hair to be cut and use the straight scissor to cut off one quarter inch. At this time gently intersect side hair with back side.

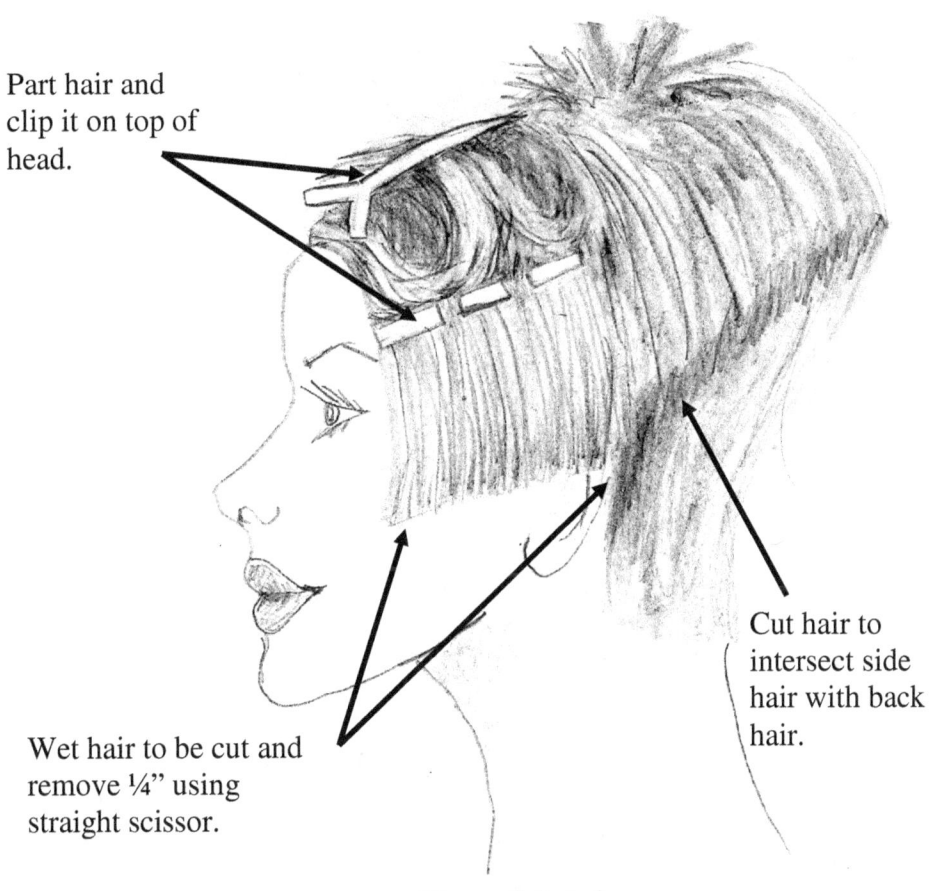

Part hair and clip it on top of head.

Cut hair to intersect side hair with back hair.

Wet hair to be cut and remove ¼" using straight scissor.

Figure 3-2 Before

NOTE

Cutting the hair ¼" shorter underneath encourages the top hair to turn under.

Figure 3-2 After shows the finished look after successfully completing Step 3.

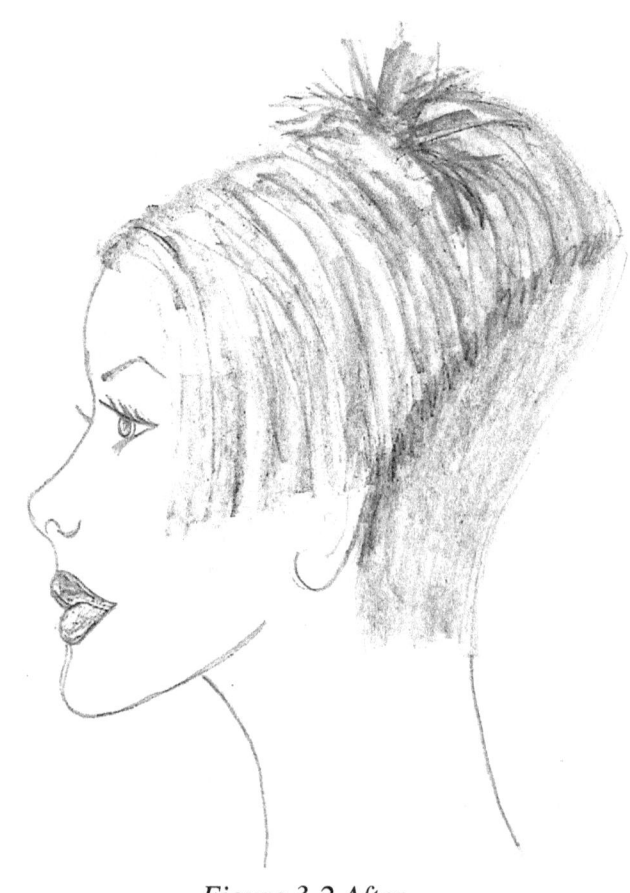

Figure 3-2 After

To encourage your hairstyle to "show itself" you should run your fingers through your hair and shake your head. This is as far as you go for now. Shaping the sides with the back is covered later in Step Five Shaping.

STEP FOUR

Cutting Spikes

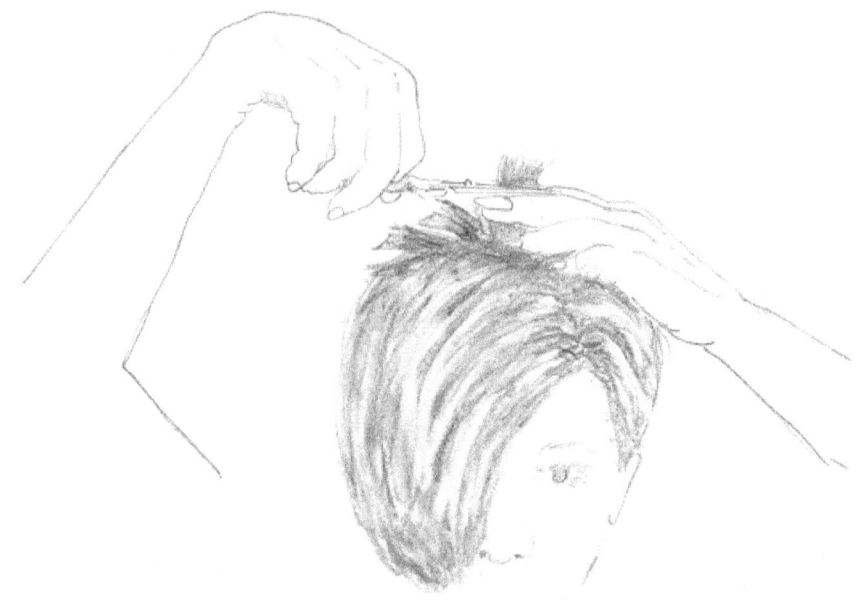

Figure 4-1

Spikes are worn toward the back of the head (the crown) to give the haircut height. Cut the spikes in the direction your hair grows. With the thinning scissor, take small sections of dry hair between your fingers as illustrated in *Figure 4-1* and cut sections leaving them 1½" - 2" long. You can cut them shorter if you prefer but remember, go slow. You can always cut more. See detail. After cutting the preferred length in the direction it is growing, take your thinning scissors and reduce the volume of the hair on one side.

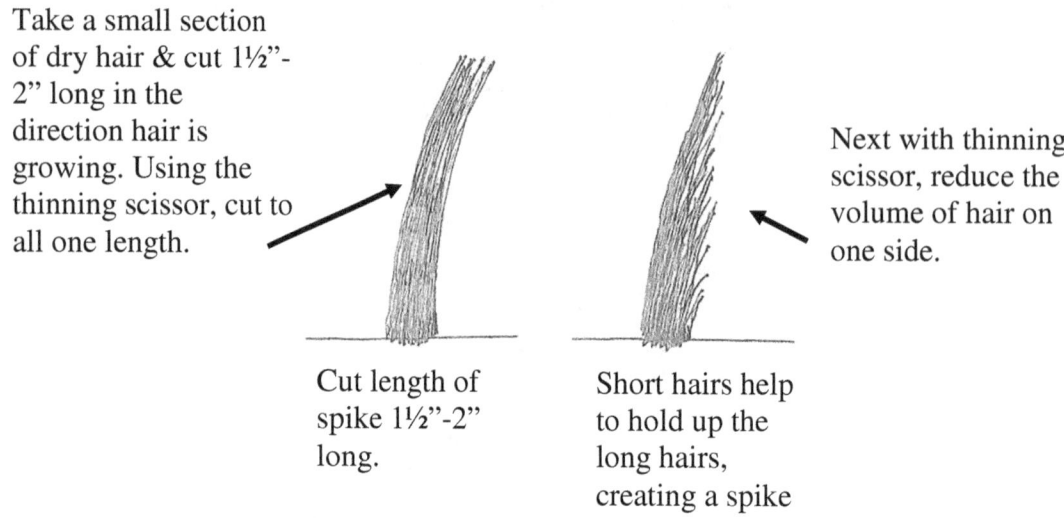

Take a small section of dry hair & cut 1½"-2" long in the direction hair is growing. Using the thinning scissor, cut to all one length.

Cut length of spike 1½"-2" long.

Next with thinning scissor, reduce the volume of hair on one side.

Short hairs help to hold up the long hairs, creating a spike

Figure 4-1 Detail

Encouraging the Spikes to Stand Up

After washing your hair, blow dry it into the desired hairstyle while running your fingers through the spiked area to create volume. At this point, when your hair is dry, lower your head and brush your hair with a nice boar bristle brush toward the floor to give your hair lots of volume and encourage the hairstyle to fall into place.

If you want more defined spiking, spray your hand with hair spray and run your fingers through the spiked area. Spraying your hand again, twist the longest hairs in your spike to create even more definition.

If you feel the spikes are not standing up enough you may need to cut a little more length off the spike as illustrated in *Figure 4-1* and *Figure 4-1 Detail*. This all depends on how much or how little spiking you desire.

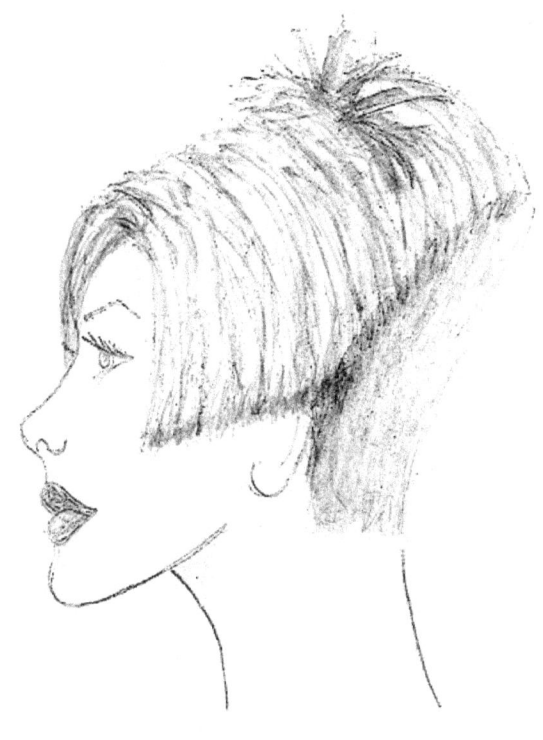

Figure 4-2

Now that you have finished the spiking, it's time to go on to Step Five Shaping. Don't be concerned if your spikes do not appear perfect yet. Letting your hairstyle "rest" for a couple of days will let you know if and where it needs tweaking.

STEP FIVE

Shaping

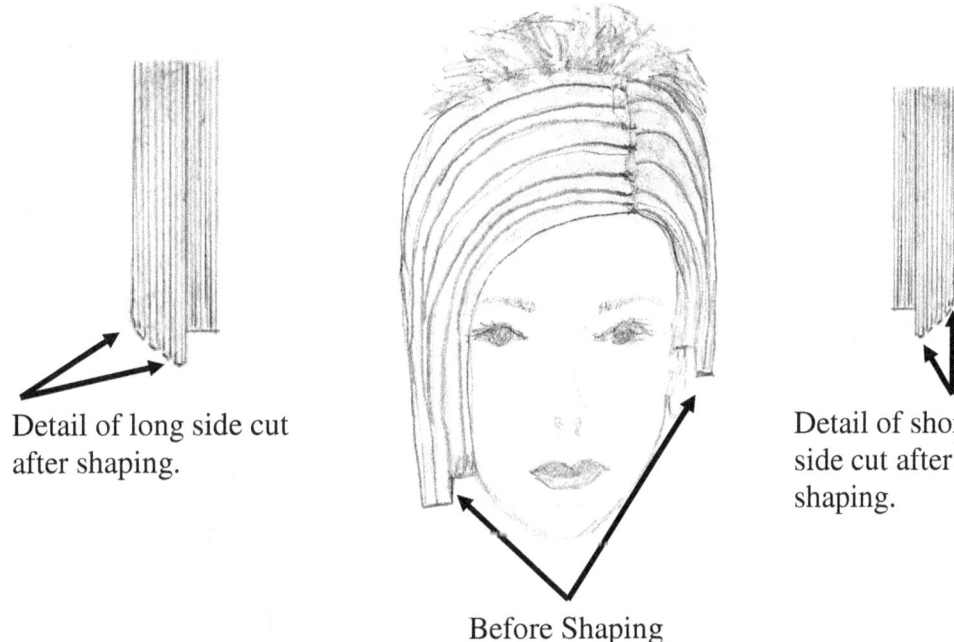

Detail of long side cut after shaping.

Detail of short side cut after shaping.

Before Shaping

Figure 5-1

Figure 5-1 (center) shows hair already cut ¼" shorter underneath on both sides (as explained in Steps 2 & 3) but before shaping. Detail illustrations (*Figure 5-1*) show outside layer after cutting to form desired shape.

Notice on *Figure 5-2* that this technique is done to help the outside hair to turn under (softly) but does not make it shorter. Look closely at *Figure 5-2*. Notice how the sides blend softly with the back. This is achieved by using the thinning scissor on dry hair and conservatively snipping surface hair to softly blend the sides and back. Do this slowly. Remember, you can always cut more.

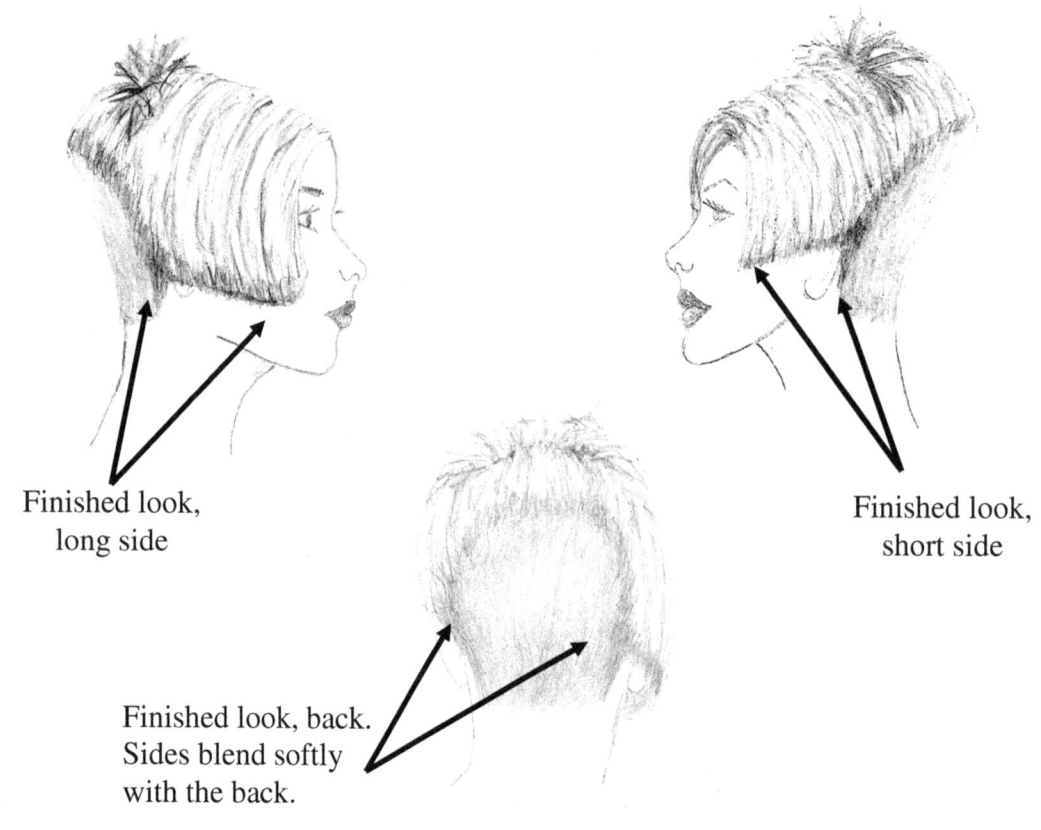

Finished look,
long side

Finished look,
short side

Finished look, back.
Sides blend softly
with the back.

Figure 5-2

After reading the instructions for *Figures 5-1 & 5-2*, you can proceed to *Figure 5-3* if you feel confidant to do so. *Figure 5-3* explains and illustrates how to achieve the finished shaping technique and shows the finished look.

Begin by using the thinning scissor on dry hair to slowly snip surface hair from cheek to earlobe on the long and short side (as shown in *Figure 5-2*) for the desired finished look.

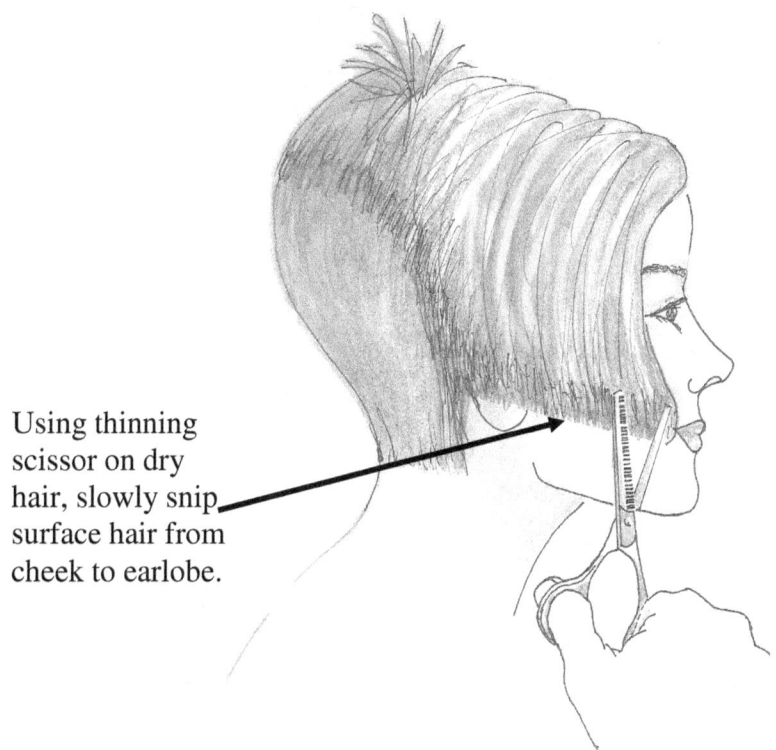

Using thinning scissor on dry hair, slowly snip surface hair from cheek to earlobe.

Figure 5-3 Long Side

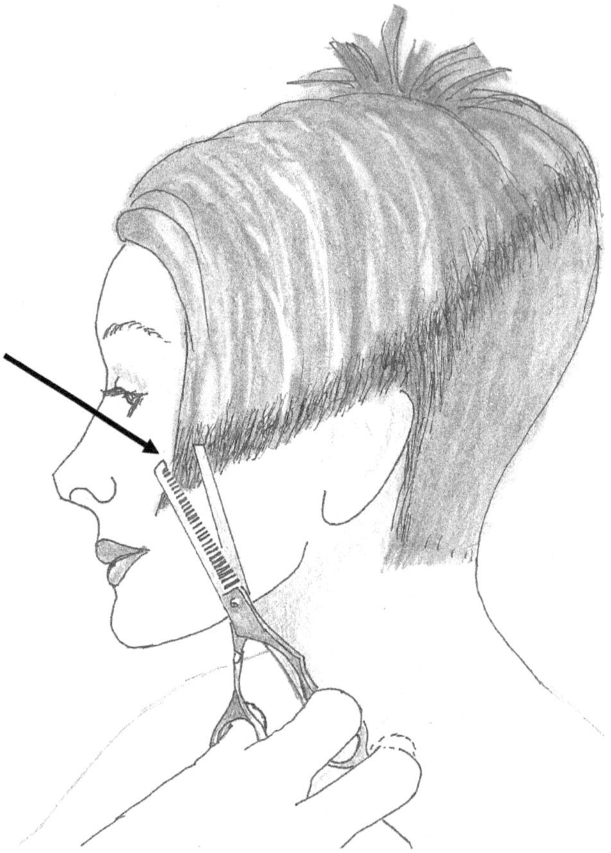

Using thinning scissor on dry hair, slowly snip surface hair from the cheek to top of the ear.

Figure 5-3 Short Side

Now that you have shaped the sides it is time to blend and shape them with the back as shown in *Figure 5-3 Back*. Earlier (in Steps 1 & 3) I suggested leaving the hair behind the ears longer. Now we are going to use that hair to make a smooth connection.

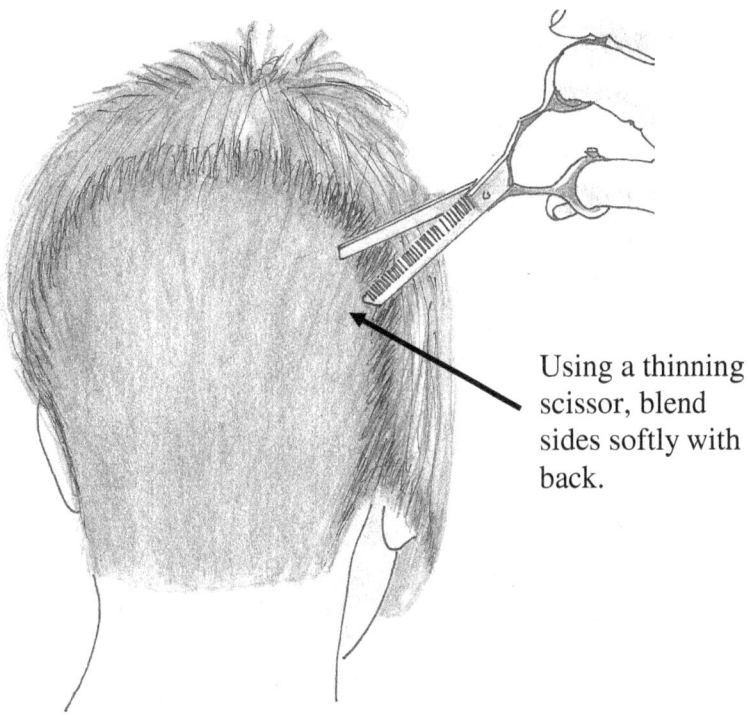

Using a thinning scissor, blend sides softly with back.

Figure 5-3 Back

While looking in the bathroom mirror use your hand mirror to blend sides softly with the back. This completes Step 5.

MAINTENANCE

If you choose to simply use this book to maintain your salon hairstyle (by learning the two simple haircutting techniques) you will still save serious money.

I recommend that you maintain your cut on a regular basis. Don't let your regular hairstyle lose its shape. Remember, your hair is constantly growing and it grows at different rates in different sections of your head. Regular maintenance makes it easier to maintain the hairstyle and will give you that salon look all the time. Remember, saving trips to the salon every 3-4 weeks is money in your pocket.

FIVE MINUTE REFRESHER

When you wear your hair short, the hair on the back of the neck is always something you need to keep looking neat. It is surprising what a positive difference this five minute refresher can make in your whole appearance.

1. Wet the back of your hair and comb it down against your neck. While looking in both the bathroom and hand mirror, use the straight scissor to cut as illustrated in *Detail 1* and *Detail 2*.

2. Using a lotion (fragrance free to prevent irritation), apply to the back of your neck and shave the neck hair as illustrated in *Detail 3*.

NOTE

Remember, if you cut your hair when it is wet, it will "shrink" up after drying. Make sure you cut a little longer than you want, to compensate. You can always cut more. Always cut dry unless otherwise noted.

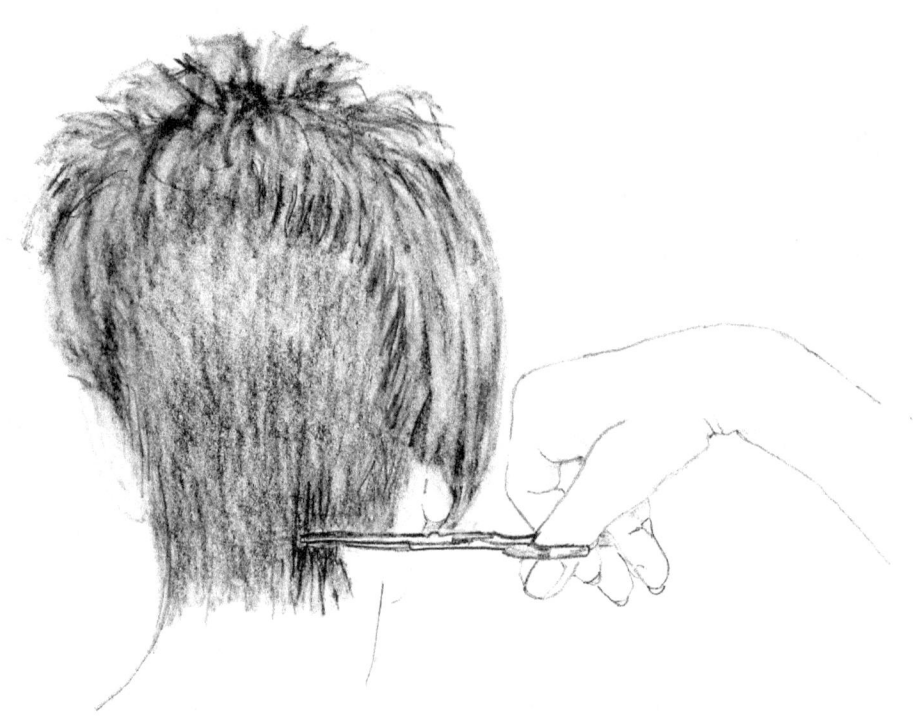

Detail 1 Before

NOTE

Wet the back of your hair and comb down against your neck. While looking in both the bathroom and hand mirror use the straight scissor to cut as illustrated in *Detail 1*.

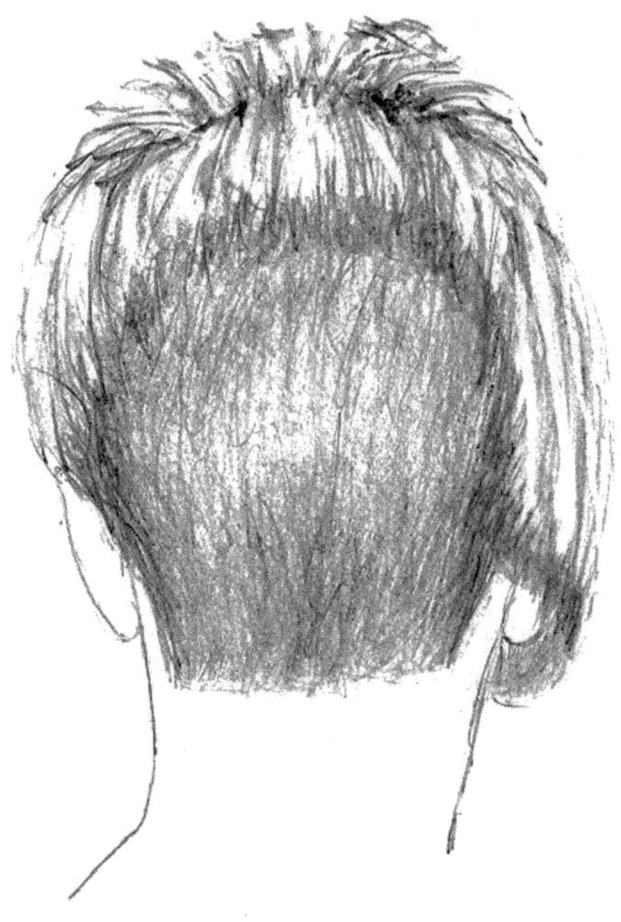

Detail 2 After

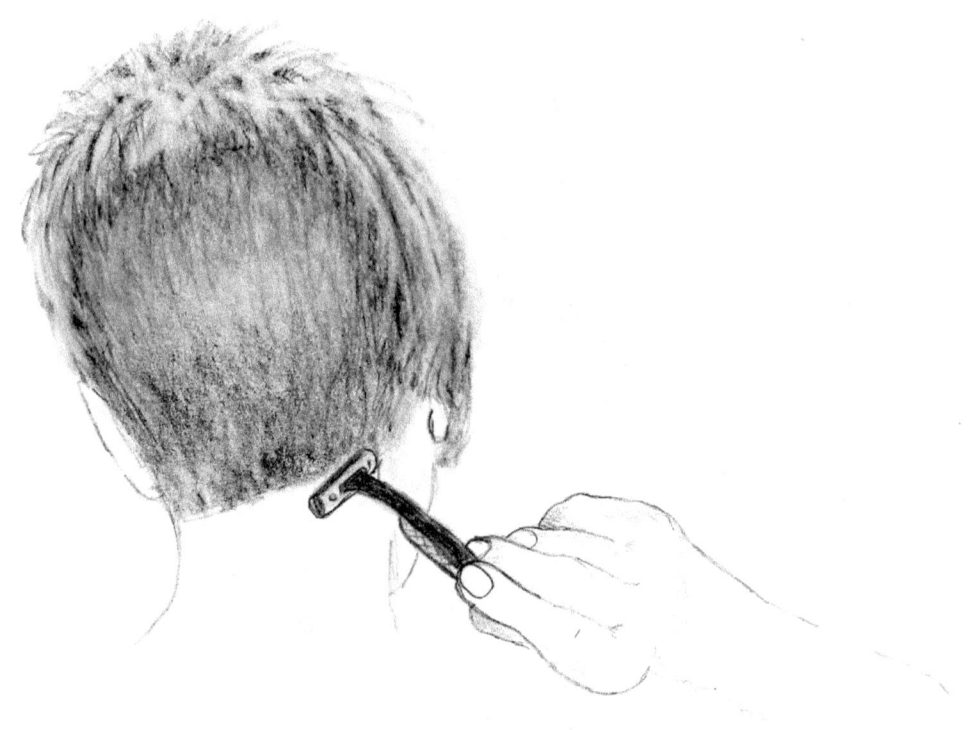

Detail 3

NOTE

Using a lotion (fragrance free to prevent irritation), apply it to the back of the neck and shave the neck hair as illustrated in *Detail 3*.

DETERMINING FACIAL SHAPES

Determining your facial shape (with the chart below) is the important first step in choosing the correct hair style for yourself. Next, will be what type of hair you have.

In general, hair is usually categorized as straight, wavy, curly or kinky. The texture can be fine, medium or thick. Also determine the volume of your hair.

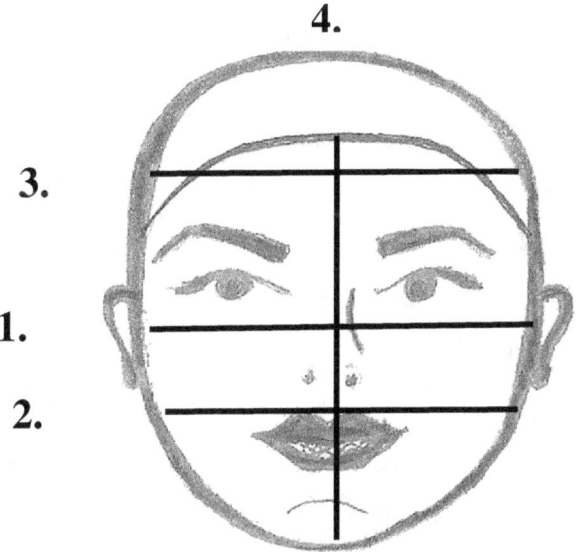

Use the diagram above and the following four steps to determine your facial shape.

1. Measure the width of your face at the top of your cheekbones. Record the result.   1. _____
2. Measure across your jaw from its widest point Record the result.   2. _____
3. Measure the widest part of your forehead (usually somewhere between the eyebrows and hairline). Record the result.   3. _____
4. Measure from your hairline to the bottom of your chin. Record the result.   4. _____

In general, the following descriptions apply to the different facial shapes:

IF YOUR FACE SHAPE IS	YOUR FACIAL SHAPE IS
Approximately as wide as it is long	Square
Approximately as wide as it is long	Round
Approximately one and a half times longer than wide	Oval
Approximately longer than it is wide	Rectangle
Narrow at the jaw line and wider at the cheekbones and/or forehead	Heart
Similar to Oval but widest at the cheekbones	Diamond
Narrow at the cheekbones and forehead and widest at the jaw line	Triangle

Your facial shape is _____

Now that you have determined your facial shape, turn to the page where your shape is displayed and read the accompanying suggestions and list them below.

Your Face Shape Suggestions:

_____
_____
_____
_____
_____
_____
_____
_____
_____
_____

Now you are ready. You have learned two simple haircutting techniques and your facial shape. Based on this information, choose the hairstyle that best suits your personality and lifestyle.

Square Shape

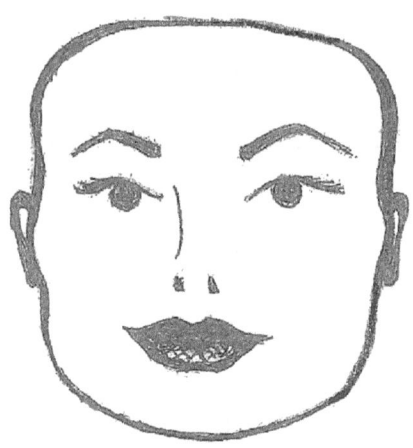

Shows a square hairline and a prominent square jaw line. For example: Katie Holmes, Sandra Bullock, Demi Moore.

Suggestions:

Keep hair at a short/medium length and include waves to create roundness about the face. Soft wispy bangs tend to soften harsh angles. Having height at the crown will lengthen the square shape. Consider a body wave. It may create a pleasant soft balance.

Stay away from styles that accentuate the sharp angles of a square facial shape. Having a straight cut at the jaw line for example, is not a good choice. You can choose a layered look as long as it stops above or below, but not at the jaw line. It's important to incorporate some roundness to your shape by increasing height at the crown or by using bangs.

Round Shape

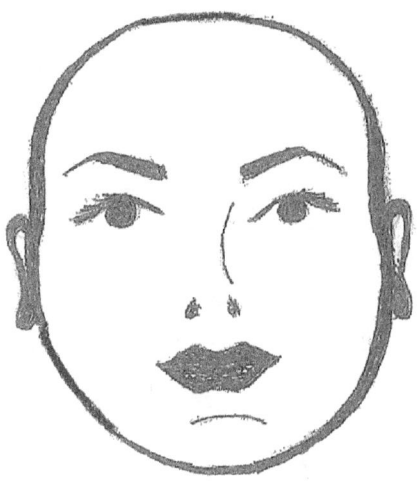

On a round face, the widest part is at the cheeks near the ears. A round chin and hairline makes for a "full" face. For example: Kate Winslet, Drew Barrymore, Ingrid Bergman.

Suggestions:

Try parting hair off-center to help reduce the roundness. Fullness at the top with some height, layering the top and having the lower part of the cut closer to your face will also give length to your face. Don't go for a short cut or straight bangs. Also stay away from styles that accentuate fullness on the sides as these will add to the rounded look.

Oval Shape

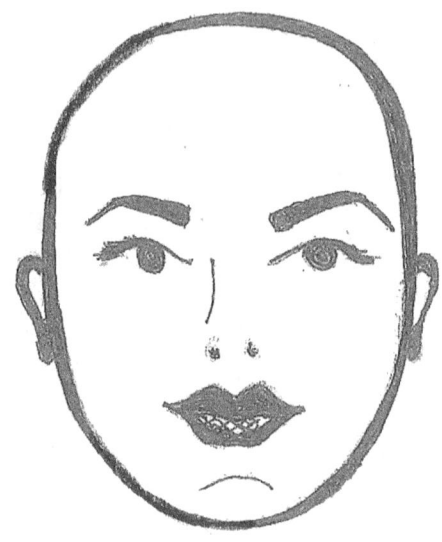

An oval shape features narrower dimensions at the jaw than at the forehead and a soft round hairline. For example: Cindy Crawford, Elle MacPherson, Julia Roberts.

Suggestions:

A very versatile shape. Will look good with almost any hairstyle. Typical shape for most models.

Because the shape is so well balanced it lends itself well to short, medium or long styles. Will look best with hair off the face.

Take advantage of the great symmetry and classic features by not having hair in the face (bangs for example). This will make the features appear other than what they are (heavier, boxy, etc.).

Rectangle Shape

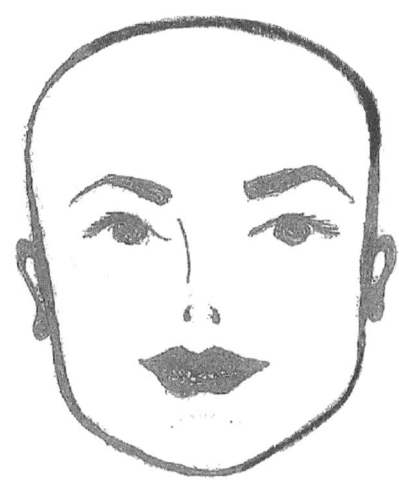

Longer than wide, this shape measures similarly at the forehead to below the cheekbones and can have a high forehead or narrow jaw at the chin. For example: Janet Jackson, Gwyneth Paltrow, Niki Taylor.

Suggestions:

Using short to medium lengths, volume at the sides and soft wispy bangs will flatter long facial shapes. This will make the face appear fuller thereby balancing the "long" look to the face. Keeping the hair length at short or medium also will shorten the length of the face. Try layering as this adds softness and diminishes the straight lines of the face.

Allowing your hair to grow long will make your face look longer. Cut down on the height. You can use center parts effectively with this facial shape. Keep hair at shoulder length or above.

Heart Shape

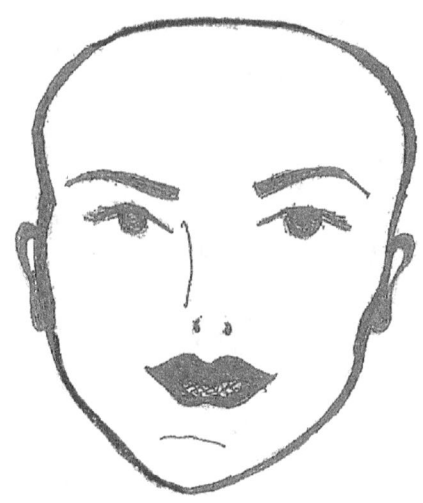

Characterized by a wide forehead and hairline narrowing down to a small chin. For example: Jennifer Love Hewitt, Lisa Kudrow, Ashley Judd.

Suggestions:

Longer hairstyles to below the jaw will flatter this shape. Also carrying hair toward the front, and off-centered parts will do well. If shorter hair is desired allow for extra volume in the back to retain balance. Shorter styles in general or too much height in the hairstyle may not be flattering.

Diamond Shape

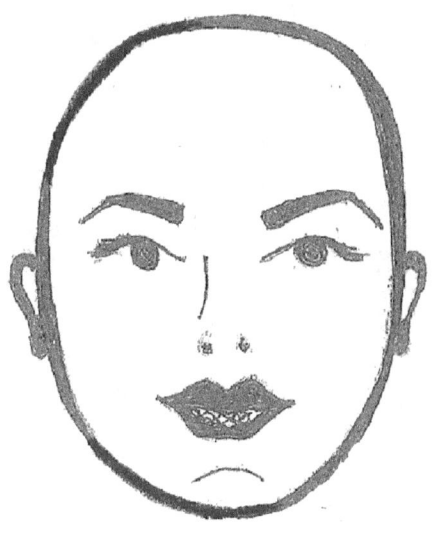

This shape is defined as wide at the cheekbones and narrow at the top and jaw. For example: Sophia Loren, Katherine Hepburn.

Suggestions:
A number of styles should work with this shape. If your shape is well-defined you may want to have volume in the back for proper balance. Don't cover your face, this shape has great features that should be exposed.

Triangle Shape

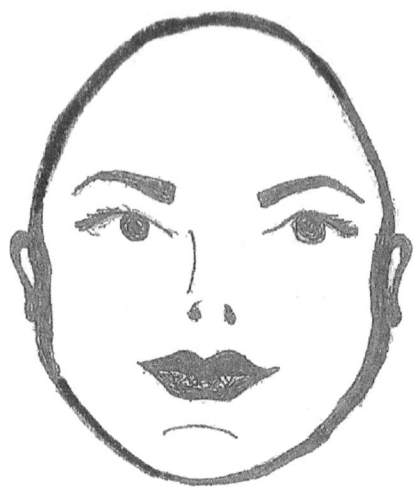

This shape is the opposite of the Heart shape. The wider part is at the jaw with the face narrowing to the top. For example: Kate Gosselin.

Suggestions:

Choose a hairstyle that is full at the forehead and narrow to the jaw. A shorter style is recommended to balance the jaw line. Layering to a full look on the top is desirable. Putting hair behind the ears will bring more attention to the eyes. Avoid center parts and long high volume hairstyles. Less volume is also recommended around the jaw. The following pages show illustrations of different hairstyles. This is to give you inspiration and get you started. They are all interchangeable with one another. Choose whatever combination works best for you.

THE IMPORTANCE OF BANGS
Make them Work for You

FOUR STYLES OF BANGS

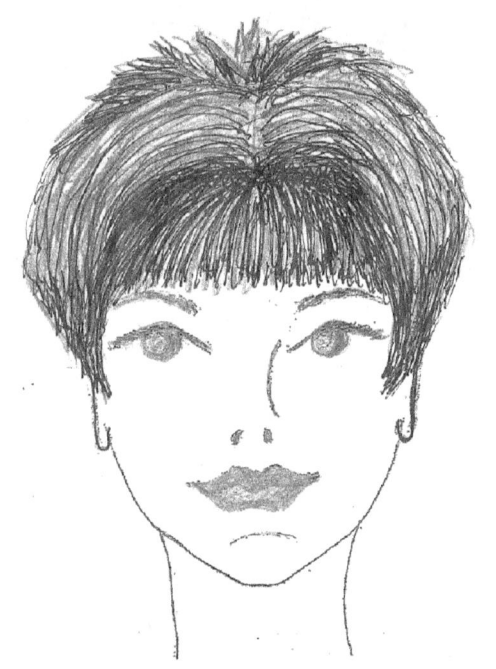 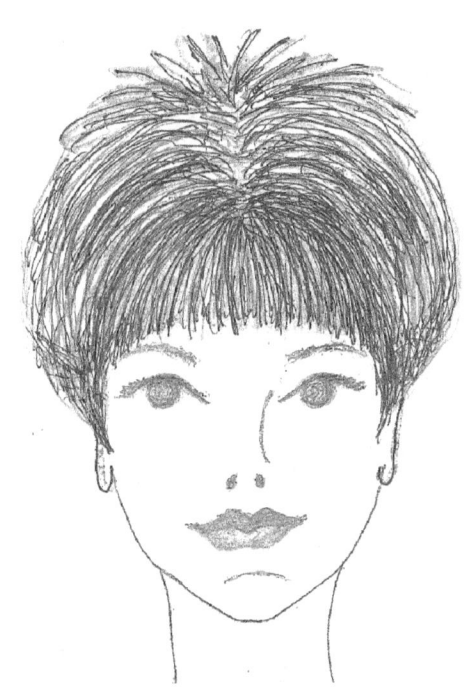

RECTANGLE   CRESCENT

The darkened areas highlight the shape of each style of bangs. After selecting the appropriate bang style for your face shape you can begin.

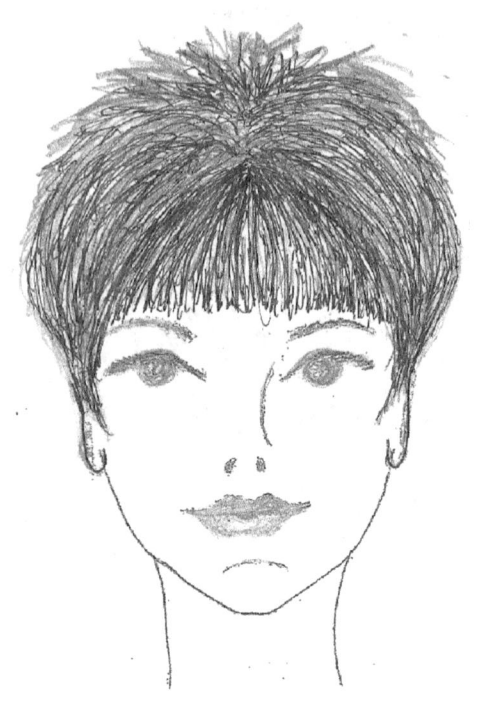
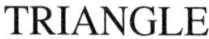
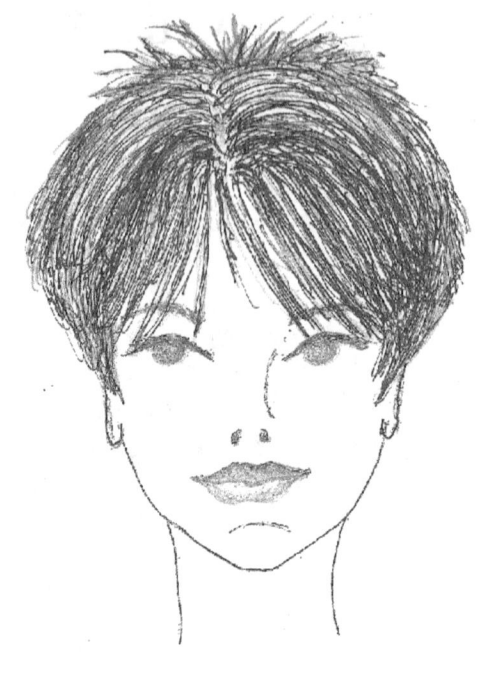

TRIANGLE   SOFT (WISPY)

Your bangs can be cut either wet or dry, whichever makes you feel more comfortable. I cut mine wet because I feel I have more control, but I also cut them longer than the desired length because when the hair dries it "shrinks" a bit. Remember, you can always cut more.

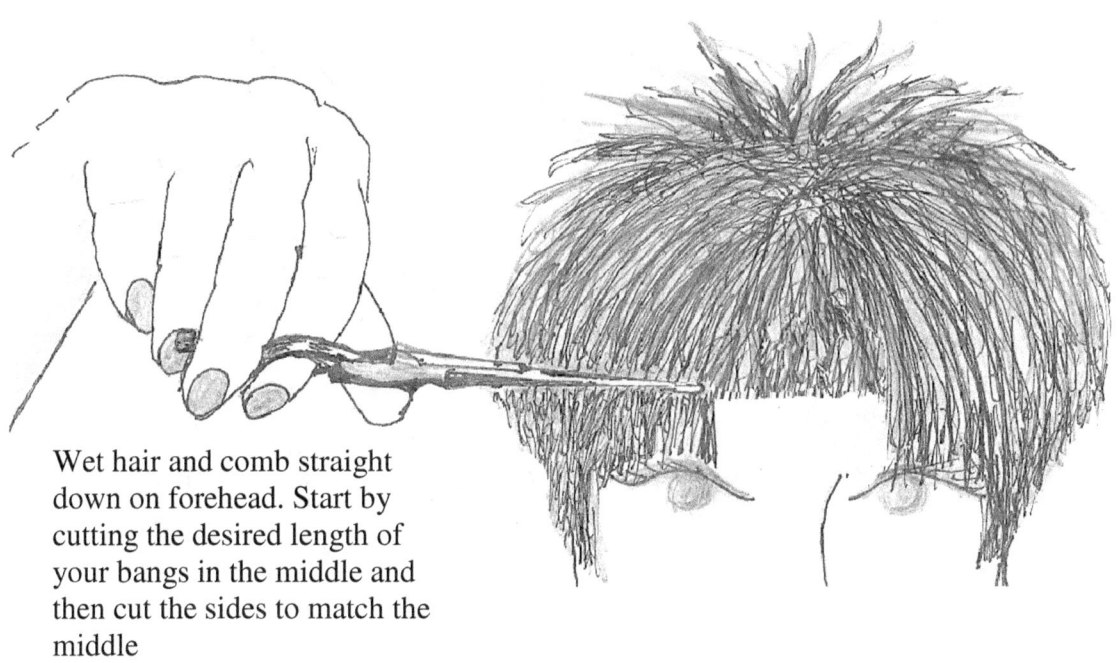

Wet hair and comb straight down on forehead. Start by cutting the desired length of your bangs in the middle and then cut the sides to match the middle

NOTE

If you cut your bangs when they are wet, cut them longer than you want to compensate for the hair shrinking after drying.

NOTE

Never attempt to cut your hair when you are in a hurry. Your full attention is needed to insure a good outcome.

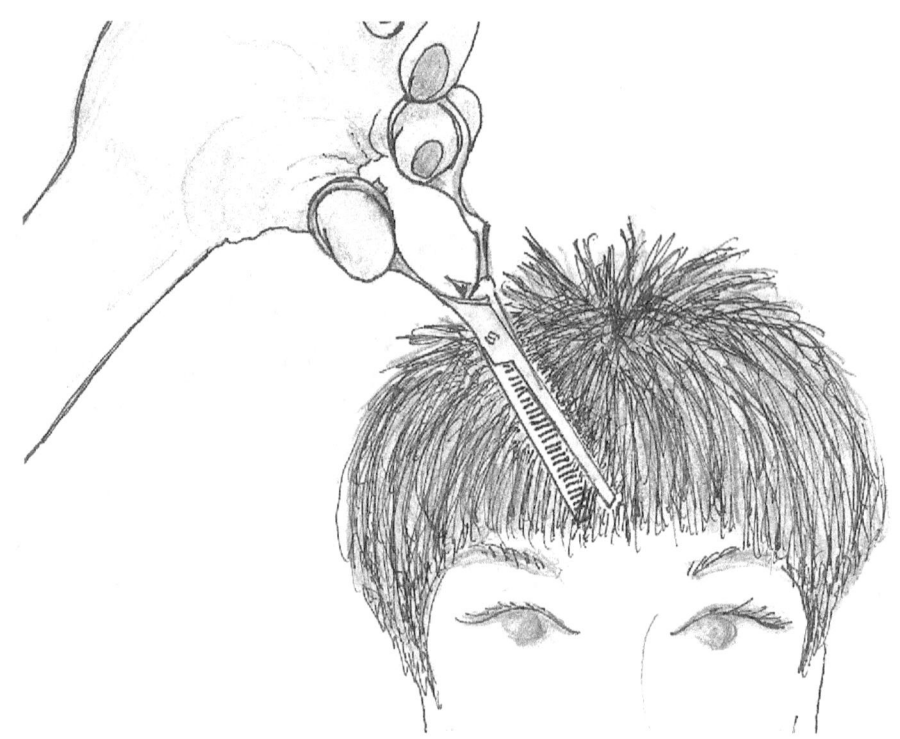

To thin your bangs or make them soft and wispy, use a thinning scissor as shown above. The thinning scissor technique can also be used for layering your hair.

MATCHING SKIN TONE
TO HAIR COLOR

Thinking of changing your hair color? Consider your skin tone also and how well the new hair color will frame your face.

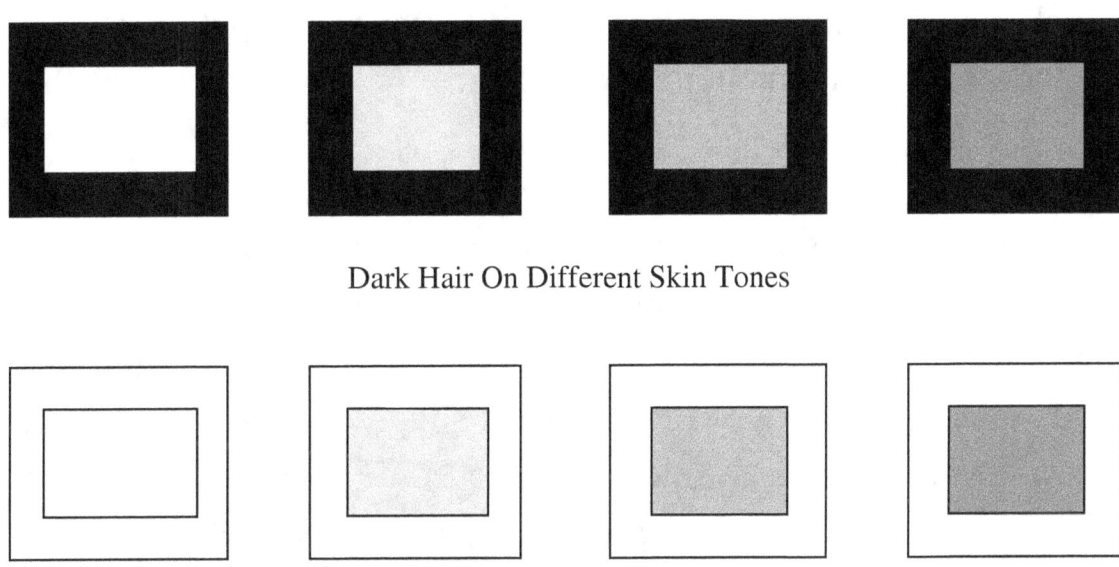

Dark Hair On Different Skin Tones

Light Hair On Different Skin Tones

The tone of your skin (lightness or darkness) and the tone of your hair color (lightness or darkness) are very important to consider when choosing hair color. This does not mean one is right and one is wrong. Just which is best suited to you when taking into consideration the softness or hardness of your look.

In my personal experience, it took time before I figured out the best color choice for myself.

My skin is light, almost unhealthy looking, and my hair is quite dark. I finally figured out that I needed to bring the two tones closer together. So I just lightened my hair (red brown tones) which made my hazel green eyes look greener and put a light self tanner on my skin which made it darker.

By doing this it brought my hair and skin tones closer together thereby creating a softer, healthier look. The lighter red-brown color also makes my eyes look greener because red (my hair) and green (my eyes) are complimentary colors. So consider your skin tone, hair color and eye color. I'm not suggesting that you try this on your own, but it is nice to have some prior idea of what direction you might want to go before consulting a professional.

TIPS FOR KEEPING YOUR HAIR LOOKING GREAT
(& Saving Money Too!)

There are many kinds of hair products for you to choose from, but this book is about DIY haircutting and saving money. With that in mind I have made a list of some alternatives that have worked well for me. I hope you find them helpful.

Help for Eliminating Bed Head
Use a silk or satin pillow case. You could buy fabric and make this pillow case yourself. Use your own pillow case as a pattern.

Help for Dry Hair
Olive oil diluted with warm water makes a great solution for this problem. Massage it into your hair and wash out with your favorite shampoo.

Help for Oily Hair
Baby powder or corn starch can be used for this problem. Sprinkle it along the scalp line and strands of hair. Brush the powder out with a boar bristle brush.

Keeping Your Hair Color from Fading

Stay out of the sun (good advice for a number of health reasons), it causes fading and dryness.

Creating Highlights

Buying a complete kit for highlighting that can only be used once is costly. I buy cream bleach. It is normally used for bleaching the hair on your arms. It is very convenient. I only mix together what I need and save the rest for next time. This is a huge saving. Follow the directions that come with the product. Place the mixture on the hair you want lightened and wrap in foil. I usually leave it on about fifteen minutes. This may not be for everyone so make sure you read the package directions and follow the test trial before using to make sure that you will not have an allergic reaction.

The following pages offer some hairstyles for inspiration that you should be able to incorporate using the tips and techniques in this book. Be creative! Here are some examples: Tomboy, Business, Glamour, Athletic, Busy Mom, etc.

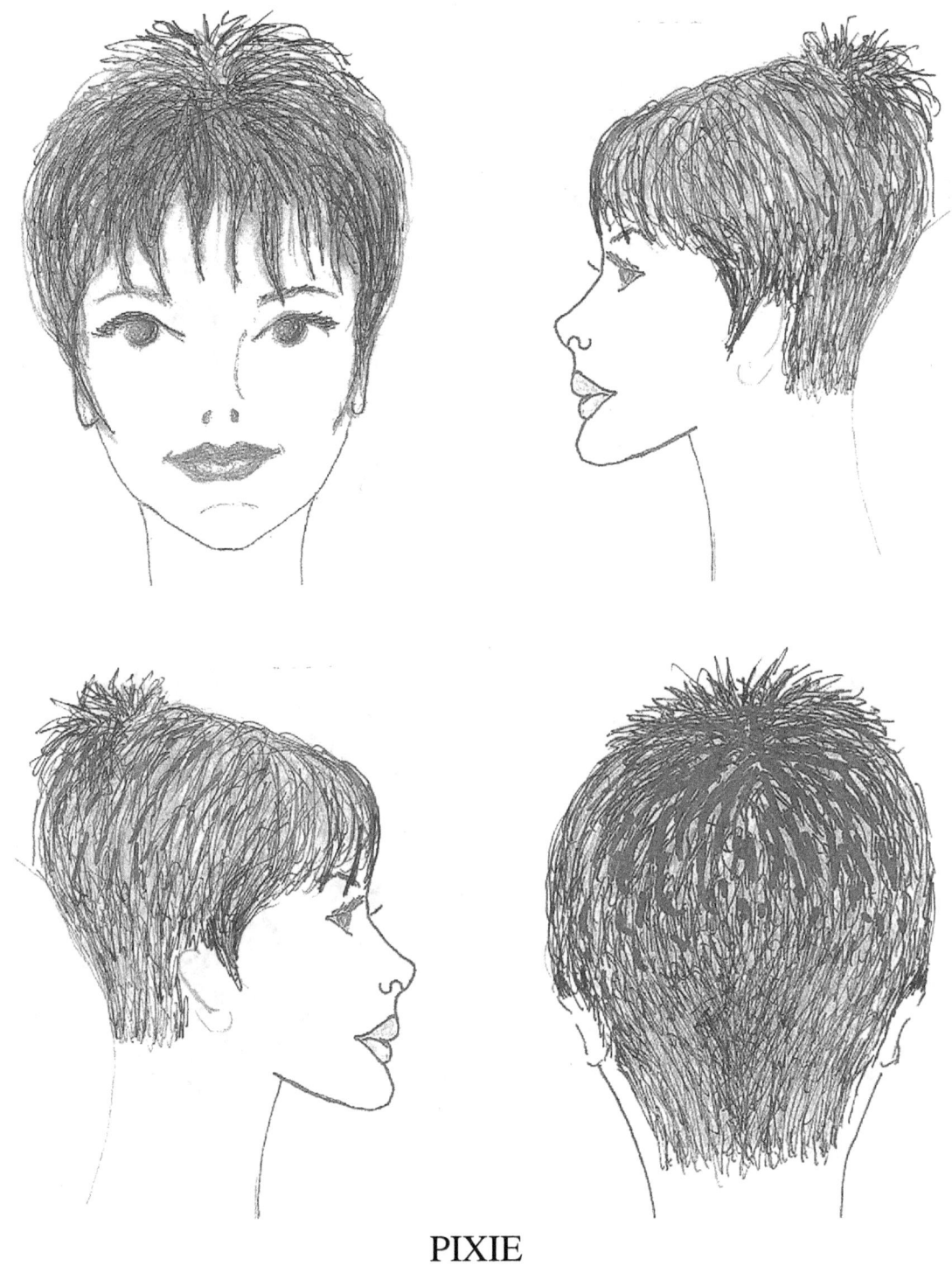

PIXIE
(Liza Minnelli)

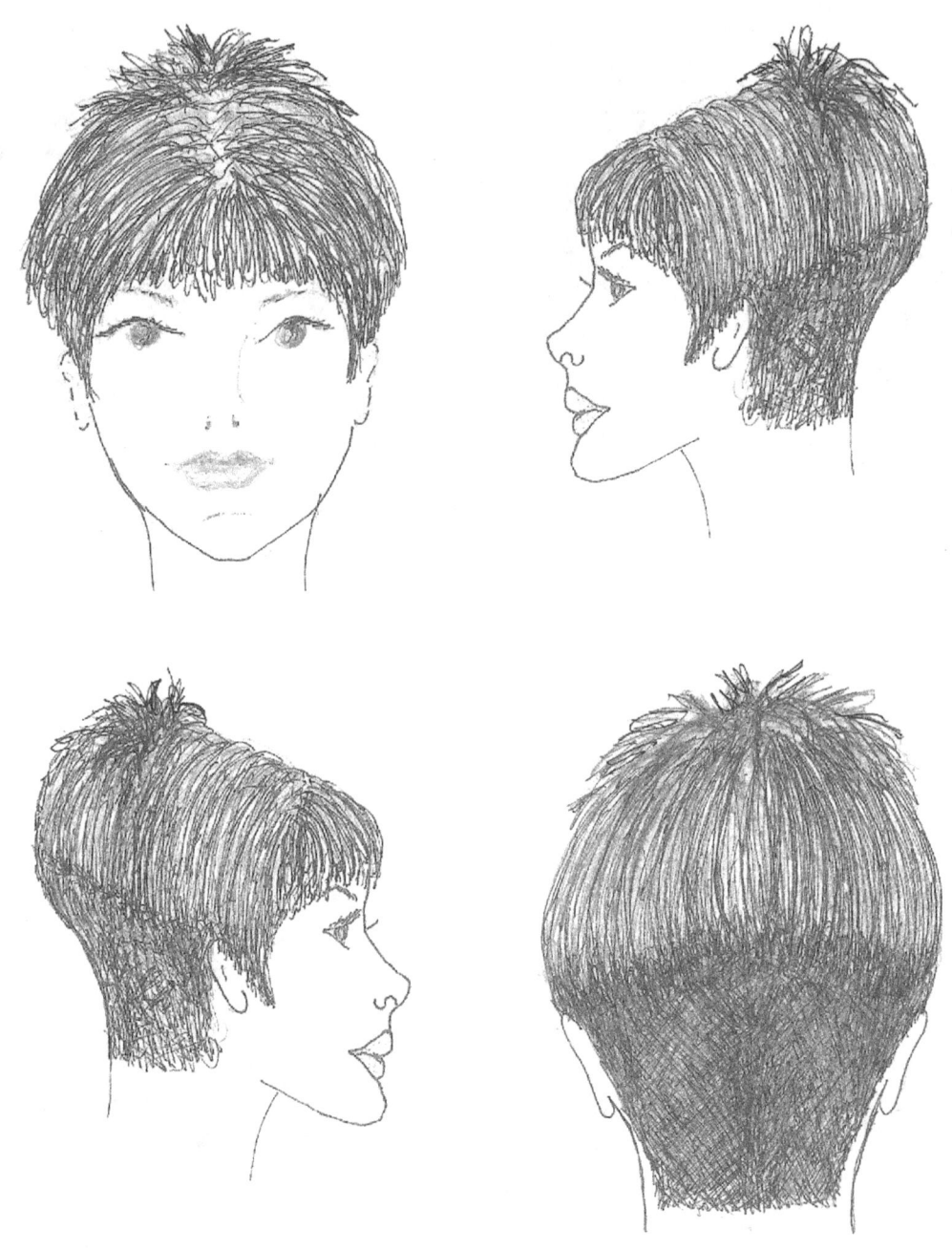

VERY SHORT

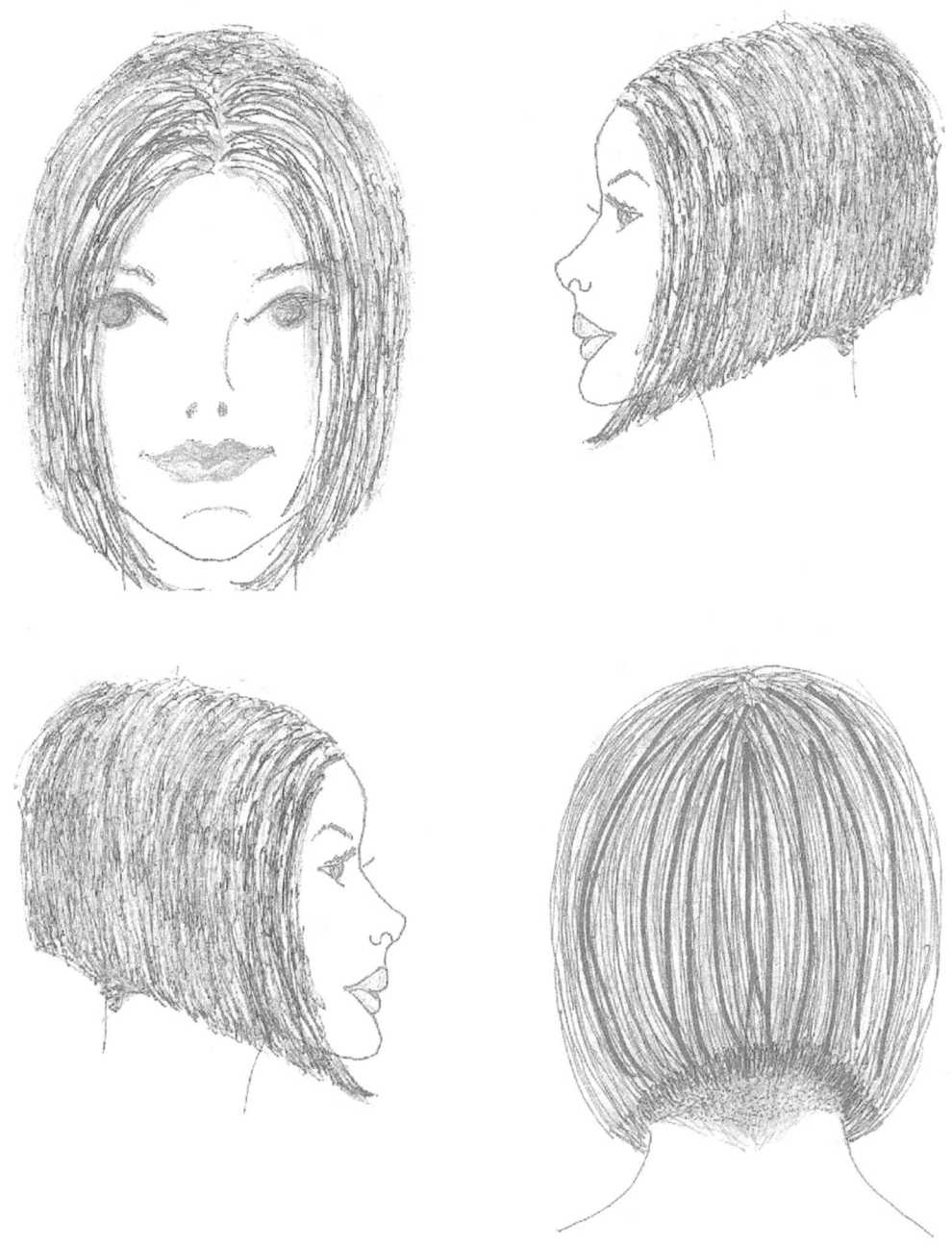

BELOW THE CHIN
(Barbra Streisand)

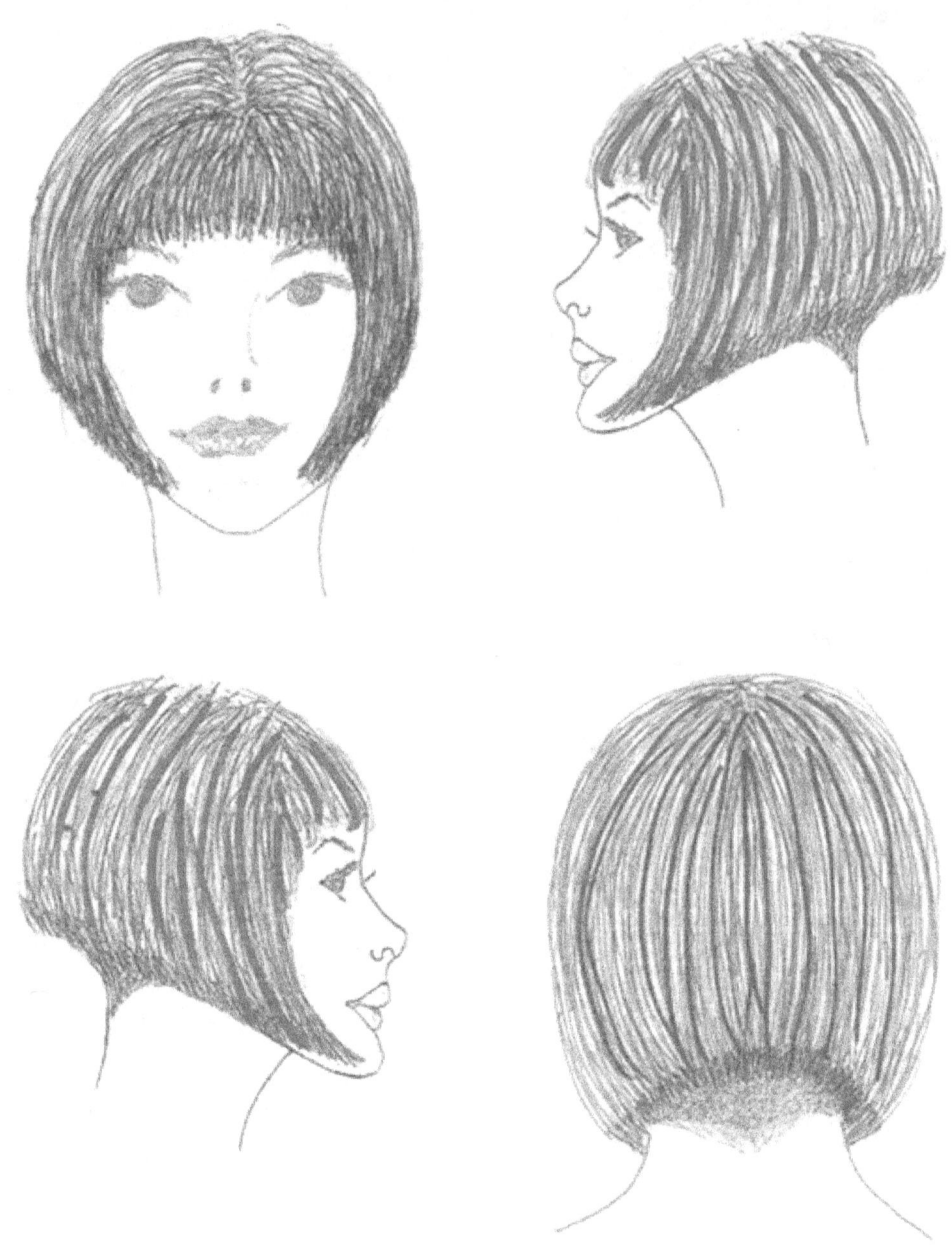

ABOVE THE CHIN
(Katie Holmes)

www.ingramcontent.com/pod-product-compliance
Lightning Source LLC
Chambersburg PA
CBHW081419280526
45788CB00009B/3166